New Abs Diet and Exercise, How to flatten your belly fat 7 Easy Steps and 7 Benefits

By
Ashlee Nicole

New Abs Diet and Exercise,
How to flatten your belly fat
7 Easy Steps and 7 Benefits

By Ashlee Nicole

Bonus Book
http://www.getspecialbonus.com/fitnessbook

Thank You For Buying This Book

I was hoping you could help your fellow book enthusiasts out and when you have a free second leave your honest feedback about this book. I certainly want to thank you in advance for doing this.

Table Of Contents

New Abs Diet and Exercise,
How to flatten your belly fat
7 Easy Steps and 7 Benefits

Introduction

One of the biggest goals of anyone interested in getting in shape is to have a flat stomach. No one wants extra body fat. You know you need to exercise and watch what you eat to flatten your belly fat, however, you also know you do not want to be in the gym for three hours everyday. Fortunately, you do not have to take up residence at your local gym to enjoy a flatter stomach. This article will go over seven steps to creating a simple diet and exercise plan that will allow you to create that flat belly you have dreamed of. It will also go over the benefits of each step so you know that you are following guidelines that are scientifically relevant, unlike the latest "Miracle Diet" infomercial you watched at 3 AM.

If you have tried a "magic pill" to flatten your abs in the past of the latest fitness gadget, you know that these items do not work. The promise of a magic pill or sculpting abs while sleeping is an empty one. In order to really achieve a toned tummy, you will have to review your diet and exercise routine.

While these steps may seem challenging at first, they are solutions that are meant to last. They are simple and sustainable tips for creating lifestyle changes that you can live with instead of unrealistic regiments that doom you to gain back the weight you lost whilst losing the abs you worked so hard to earn. The seven steps you will need to include in your ab flattening routine start by having you identify why you want to make changes to your routine. They also include steps related to your nutrition plan so you can eat to fuel your body without feeling deprived. Finally, the remaining steps are dedicated to helping you create a simple and effective exercise routine.

When starting this routine you will need to purchase a few items. Most will be the healthy foods you will want to use to fuel your body. While you won't need to join a gym or buy a lot of equipment, there are a few items that you might be interested in purchasing. Read over each section to see what you will want to start with. However, you definitely will want to invest in a journal. If you do not have flat abs now you will need to make some changes and until you accurately document your current habits, you will not find success in the future.

Are you ready to take on this challenge and change yourself from flab to fab? We promise that you will be successful if you follow these tips. Read on to uncover the seven steps and get started on your personal transformation today.

Step 1: Identifying your "Why?"

To make any lasting lifestyle change, you need to first identify why you want to make that change. This step applies to getting flat abs as much as is does to any other goals you want to reach. Before you start trying to implement the changes that will help you sculpt a more toned mid-section, you have to understand why you want to make these changes.

It does not matter what your reason is, but your reason needs to matter to you. Once you are clear on why you want to start this plan, write this reason down and make it visible. Set it as the background on your phone, create e-mail reminders that mention your reason for committing to your plan, do anything and everything to make your motivation for achieving your new physique hard to avoid.

Benefit of Identifying your "Why?"

Unless you only want to enjoy your flat abs for a month after earning them, you will have to make a lifestyle change. The benefit of identifying you "why," is that you'll be able to make your change permanent. Lifestyle changes are not based on willpower. Rather they are based on making small changes that become habits.

Psychology tells us that there are five stages of a lasting behavior change. These experts have found that unless you are emotionally connected to your reasons to implement a lifestyle changes, you will not be able to make this change into a habit. Spending time identifying your "why?" will go a long way in ensuring your abs last for more than one beach season. Take the time to identify your why before attempting to try any other step.

Step 2: Reviewing your current nutrition plan.

Once you know why you want to work on that six-pack, you will need to start making changes to your current nutrition plan. The saying "abs are made in the kitchen," has a lot of truth to it. Without properly fueling your body and your workouts, you won't have the energy you need to see results.

The first step in making any changes to your diet is reviewing your current nutrition plan. If you are like most people, you probably do not even know what you eat each day. Take time to take stock of what are eating. Keep a food log or make things easier by snapping photos of your intended meals. Review your actions at the end of each day for one week and record any particularly destructive food choices. Try to identify why you made these choices so you can take steps to avoid making them in the future.

Benefit of Reviewing your Current Nutrition Plan

You cannot make changes to your plan until you know what you are actually eating. By logging your meals, the time you eat these foods, and identifying potential destructive patterns, you will be able to identify possible solutions. If you dip into the candy bowl at work every time you pass the break room, you could be adding an extra 300 calories or more each day and a half a pound to the number on the scale each week. Become aware of a pattern like this, and you can prevent it. For example, carrying around a water bottle can help you keep your hands occupied. Taking a swig of water can substitute mindless candy eating. Finding small ways to change your nutrition plan for the better is impossible if you do not know what are eating right now. You must identify your current eating habits if you are going to make new eating habits that address your needs.

Step 3: Getting a Handle on Proper Nutrition

One you have identified your current eating habits and any obvious issues, you will need to make changes to ensure your diet is in line with your fitness goals. To create a nutrition plan that will give you results you will need to modify the calories you consume, your portion sizes, and the type of foods you are eating. In this section we will review general guidelines for each of these aspects of your ideal flat belly diet. Make these changes incrementally and your "diet" will be more of a lasting lifestyle change than a deprivation plan.

The number of calories you need to consume will depend on your height, weight, gender, and activity level. One common mistake that dieters make is eating too few calories. Men should never eat fewer than 1500 calories and women should never eat less than 1200 calories. If you aren't sure the amount of calories that is right for you try this free resource: http://www.choosemyplate.gov/myplate/index.aspx

Unless you buy only prepackaged foods, you will not be able to properly track the number of calories you are consuming without knowledge of portion sizes. This will be especially important when you eat at a restaurant. Many restaurants serve portions so large that you could end up consuming more than your daily calorie needs in a single meal. For example, a single serving of lean protein is four ounces and around 160 calories. However, order a burger at a restaurant and you could end up with a whole pound of meat and at least four times the calories.

When logging meals and calories, several visual guidelines are useful. A deck of cards is the size of four ounces of meat. A tablespoon serving is about the size of a poker chip. A baseball is about the size of one cup. Many other analogies can be found online that may relate more to items in your daily life. However, having a basic understanding of these portions can be invaluable when you are dining on the go and trying to achieve flat abs.

Finally, you will want to make sure the quality of your calories is appropriate. There are three main types of fuel that our bodies consume: carbohydrates, proteins, and fats. Out of your daily calories, around half should come from a carbohydrate fuel source, slightly more than a quarter from a protein fuel source, and the remaining quarter from fats. Alcohol is another source of calories that must be consumed in moderation. Limit your consumption of alcohol to avoid empty calories and the temptation to eat additional food calories.

Keep in mind that not all carbohydrates, proteins, and fats are created equal. Carbohydrates from fruits, vegetables, and non-refined breads are much healthier than those from refined sources and packaged foods. Lean sources of proteins like chicken, fish, and beans should take up more of your protein calories than those from beef and other higher fat sources. Fats from packaged foods should be limited, however, healthy fats such as those found in olive oil, fish, and flax seeds are needed in the body.

Benefits of Getting a Handle on Proper Nutrition:

To get flat abs, you need to have a low body fat percentage. While exercise is important, you cannot completely undo bad eating habits by working out. This is why it is important to fuel your body properly if you want to enjoy a flatter stomach.

Counting calories and understanding how many calories you are consuming by monitoring meal portion sizes is important to make sure you are properly fueling your body. If you do not follow the recommended caloric intake for your gender, weight, and activity level, you could do damage to your body. While creating a large calorie deficit will give you weight loss results the first week or too, you will ultimately end up putting your body into starvation mode if you continue this pattern.

If your body is in starvation mode you won't be able to lose weight and you will wreck havoc on your metabolism. Even if you do not eat enough calories, your body needs to get its energy somewhere. Decide not to properly fuel your body and it will break down its own tissues for fuel. Do not make this rookie mistake! Following the resource mentioned above is a great place to start. Creating a guideline that fits your personal needs. You can also monitor your overall weight loss to make sure you are eating enough calories. If you are losing more than two to half a pound of weight each week (after the first month) you are not reaching your goals in a sustainable way. The benefit of following these guidelines is that you will enjoy weight loss and flat abs for life if you work on it at the proper pace for your body.

Make sure you are fueling you body with enough but not too much food and the right types of food. Many people try to avoid eating carbohydrates. However, carbohydrates are the main source of energy for the entire body and most importantly the brain. If you have ever tried to restrict carbohydrates you already know this because you probably had a hard time thinking clearly on this diet. Fueling your body properly will not only help you enjoy a better overall physique, but it will allow you to avoid diseases such as cancer and diabetes.

Step 4: Creating a Complete Exercise Routine

Once you have gone through the first three steps, you will need to create a complete exercise routine. A solid exercise routine includes three key components: cardiovascular fitness, strength training, and flexibility. Each component is needed to help you lose weight and ultimately, reveal those tight abs.

Benefit of Creating a Complete Exercise Routine:

Many people think that just doing thousands of crunches or other abdominal exercises every day, will result in toned, flat abs. The reality is that spot reduction, the idea that you can complete an exercise for one body part to completely tone that area, is a myth. A flat ab routine requires a well-rounded overall exercise routine. You need a low body fat percentage to achieve flat abs and that comes from diet and a complete exercise routine, not just crunches!

Step 5: Setting Up Your Cardiovascular Fitness Routine

If you have more than ten pounds to lose, your cardiovascular routine will be very important to eliminating the excess body fat that is covering your abdominal muscles. Any type of exercise that raises your heart rate counts as cardiovascular fitness. Examples include walking, running, biking, and swimming. Find the exercise that you enjoy the most to ensure that you will stick with your plan. Start by completing this exercise a minimum of thirty minutes three days a week. Gradually work up to completing cardiovascular sessions up to six days a week. If you complete a low intensity activity such as walking, you will need to complete at least two and a half hours each week. However, if you can advance to a higher intensity activity, such as running, you can reduce your minimum overall cardiovascular training commitment to one and a half hours each week.

If you have not exercised in a while, it is important to see a doctor for clearance and to gradually increase the duration of your cardiovascular fitness sessions. However, studies have shown that breaking sessions down into 10 or 15 minute time periods is as beneficial to weight loss and overall health as completing one thirty minute session all at once. Look at your schedule at the beginning of the week and write in when you will work out at the beginning of the week so you get your workouts in even if they are shorter in duration.

When you are done with your cardiovascular routine, complete basic stretches for each major muscle group to help prevent injury. You will want to hold each stretch for a minimum of 20 seconds. Aim to repeat each stretch a minimum of two times per muscle. You can stretch daily and may want to add a day of yoga to your fitness routine to really help you focus on flexibility training.

Benefits of Setting Up Your Cardiovascular Fitness Routine

Cardiovascular fitness increases your heart rate and this is a benefit because it will cause your body to burn more calories. To get flat abs you will need to lose weight and to lose weight you need to burn calories. If you reduce your calorie intake by 250 calories each day (about what's in a personal size M&M candy bag) and increase your calorie output by 250 calories a day (completing a cardiovascular activity for for about 30 minutes) you can expect a one pound weight loss each week. Finally, cardiovascular training increases the health of your heart. A healthy heart will prevent heart disease and side effects such as high blood pressure. This form of fitness can save you hundreds of dollars each year by keeping you off of blood pressure and other medications.

Stretching at the end of your cardiovascular fitness routine helps increase the range of motion around your joints. In this way, flexibility training can help you prevent injuries. Staying healthy is important if you want to keep up with your exercise plan. Practicing Yoga is a great way to work on this aspect of your fitness and to help you be more mindful as the practice closes with mediation. If you are stressed, it is harder for your body to lose weight.

Step 6: Strength Training Routine Set-Up

In addition to finding a heart pumping activity to complete most days of the week, you will need to create a strength training routine. Strength training exercises involve adding resistance to the muscles of the body. Resistance used in strength training may come from free weights (dumbbells), resistance bands, medicine balls, weight machines, or even your own body weight. No matter what props you use, the goal of strength exercises will be to increase the fitness of your muscles.

Working with a personal trainer is the best way to create a basic strength training routine that will work for your needs. However, there are some key points that we will review here. Strength training should be completed at least 2 days a week and up to 3 days a week. Starting with 2 days a week is fine for a beginner and will increase your muscular fitness 80% as much as a 3-day training plan. No matter how many days are included in your routine, a solid plan will give muscles 48 hrs of rest between sessions. If you do not have time to complete a full body strength training routine 2-3times a week in addition to your cardiovascular routine, you may want to work upper body muscles one day and lower body muscles the following day. As long as you aren't working the same muscles two days in a row, this plan is fine.

When strength training, you will want to complete 2-3 sets of each exercise in your plan. A good plan will include 8-10 exercises, one for each major muscle group. The major muscles to work are: chest, back, abs, shoulders, triceps, biceps, hamstrings, quadriceps, glutes (butt muscles), and calves. Use a weight for each exercise that allows you to complete 10-15 reps before you need a rest. If you can complete more than 15 reps, you need to increase the weight you are using. Constantly monitor your workout so you are always challenging your body and getting closer to those tight abs.

Benefit of Setting Up Your Strength Training Fitness Routine

Strength training is an important part of your flat stomach training routine, because it increases your muscle tone. Muscle tissue burns more calories at rest than fat or other body tissues. By incorporating strength training in your fitness routine, you will increase your body's resting metabolism. This means that even when you are sitting around watching TV you will be burning more calories than you would without this muscle tone. The more calories you burn, the more weight you will lose. To achieve flat abs you need a low body fat percentage and increasing your lean (muscular) body weight is crucial if you want to get reach your goal.

Step 7: Including the Correct Abdominal Exercises

On strength training days you will want to include abdominal exercises. However, some exercises are better than others. Traditional crunches are not even the list of the top ten most effective exercises for abs!

Which ab exercises should you do? Stay away from weight machines and the traditional crunch. Instead practice the bicycle crunch, captains chair crunch, stability (or swiss ball) crunch, and plank to maximize your time at the gym. A personal trainer can help make sure you are doing each exercise with the proper form.

Finally, keep in mind that many exercises use your abs without you even knowing it! The push-up does not focus on the abdominal muscles; however, it requires strong abs if you complete it correctly. Compound fitness moves such as those that use a medicine ball also require strong abdominal muscles. As soon are you are able to have good enough form to stop using the weight machines at the gym, try to use dumbbells and other props that require you to engage your abs to get the most efficient workout.

Benefit of Including the Correct Abdominal Exercises

Many people incorrectly think that they can shape their abs just by doing abdominal muscle exercises. The truth is you cannot spot reduce an area on your body and you must incorporate cardiovascular training and an overall strength training plan to see real results. However, your abs are muscles and sculpting the ab muscles you have will have them burning calories while you are resting just as much as your biceps will. Making sure you select the correct abdominal exercises ensures that you see a benefit as a result of your time at the gym. The bicycle crunch activates the abdominal muscles about 150% more than a traditional crunch.

Conclusion:

Having flat abs you can show off at the beach requires a knowledge of nutritional and physical activity guidelines. While there is no magic pill that will get you flat abs, if you follow the seven steps we have shared in this article, you can see results without needing to spend hours at the gym. The most important step to flat abs is the first step, understanding your "why." If you do not have a reason to start your ab flattening lifestyle change, you won't be able to exchange these healthy habits for the old ones.

While the seven steps we discussed may seem challenging to incorporate in one day, starting with small changes will go a long way in helping you create the abs you dream of. If you take small steps to make changes, you will make your flatter abs part of your lifestyle instead of a temporary phase.

When you have flat abs, you will also have a narrow waist. One of the biggest indicators of someone at risk for a heart attack is a high waist to hip ratio. Working on getting sculpted abs will not only make you the envy of your friends, but it will also ensure you are living a healthy lifestyle.

Special Bonus Book for buying this book:
Bonus Book

www.ingramcontent.com/pod-product-compliance
Lightning Source LLC
Chambersburg PA
CBHW080359290526
45791CB00009BA/2929